EI

EAT BETTER

The Ultimate Guide to Healthy Eating, Learn About Nutrition and What Eating Healthy is All About and Tips on Planning Healthy Meals for You and Your Family

Descrierea CIP a Bibliotecii Naţionale a României
ELEANOR TEVIN
EAT BETTER. The Ultimate Guide to Healthy Eating, Learn About Nutrition and What Eating Healthy is All About and Tips on Planning Healthy Meals for You and Your Family / Eleanor Tevin – Bucharest: Editura My Ebook, 2021
ISBN

ELEANOR TEVIN

EAT BETTER

The Ultimate Guide to Healthy Eating, Learn About Nutrition and What Eating Healthy is All About and Tips on Planning Healthy Meals for You and Your Family

My Ebook Publishing House
Bucharest, 2021

TABLE OF CONTENTS

INTRODUCTION

Everyone knows that there is something that they could change in their life to become healthier. For most people, it's getting more exercise and eating a healthier diet. But, how do you know if you are eating healthy or not? There are so many different diets and strategies on the market, how do you know what to do?

This eBook is designed to provide you with some basic guidelines to become a healthy eater as well as some tips on how to begin changing your eating habits. For example, breakfast is incredibly important and many people don't give it its due. You need to eat breakfast to literally "break the fast." Unfortunately, many people skip breakfast and they are so hungry by the time lunch comes around that they eat like they've never eaten before. Then they have a slump and want to take a nap. Eating healthy and with good eating habits can solve these typesof problems.

Being a healthy eater requires that you become educated and smart about what you put in your mouth. You really are what you eat, so if you eat a lot of fats, well, you know what happens. However, being food smart doesn't mean that youhave to learn all of these different calorie-counting strategies or that you have to study labels. Healthy eating is about balance and moderation.

This eBook is your guide to learning to eat healthy and how to balance out yourmeals. It will show you how you can eat healthy, lose weight and begin to havea better overall feeling of healthiness in your life. This doesn't mean that you have to give up your favorite foods, but you will learn how to make your favoritefoods part of a healthy lifestyle.

Chapter 1

Eating for a Healthier You

Most people know they need to improve their diets in one way or another. They also recognize how difficult this is when you drive down the street and you see a McDonald's on every corner or a line of fast food restaurants. Our lives have all become about convenience and in exchange for convenience we have become the most obese country in the world. With our instant gratification lifestyles we also know that eating healthy can be a challenge. However, it doesn't have to be this way and there are steps that you can take to balance out your life so that you can enjoy a Happy Meal with the kids on occasion.

Making your everyday diet healthier will allow you to improve the way you look, as well as the way you think. It's never too late to change your eating habits, you just have to have the personal motivation to do it.

Is Your Diet Healthy Enough?

Everyone wants a healthier diet, but with all of the conflicting nutrition information in the media it is hard to determine what type of diet is healthy. There are many factors that contribute to a healthy diet. It is important to evaluate the current diet that you eat before you embark on a plan to become ahealthier eater.

Begin by asking yourself these simple questions:

1. **Do I eat a variety of different foods?**Variety is one of many important parts of a healthy diet. It is important to eat foods from all ofthe food groups. If you find yourself avoiding certain food groups, such as fruits and vegetables, then it may be time to adjust the way you eat.

2. **Do I eat fruits and vegetables?** It is important to choose from a variety of different fruits and vegetables. In fact, you want to get all ofthe different colors of these foods in your diet because each offers their own unique vitamins and minerals that are essential to your diet.Eat dark greens, reds, oranges and yellows.

3. **Do I eat breakfast?**The absence of breakfast is a good indicator that you are not eating very healthy. If you don't eat breakfast you need tobegin working on that aspect of your diet, as your body may think that it's starving.

4. **Do I choose low fat foods over high fat foods?** There are low fat alternatives in a variety of foods including all dairies and meats. A great way to avoid a lot of fat is to prepare your own meals instead ofeating prepared foods such as TV dinners.

5. **Do I drink a lot of water?** Water is the foundation to life. Your body needs plenty of water and is important for maintaining a healthy diet. If you drink a lot of soda or coffee, you may be dehydrating yourself.

6. **Am I able to maintain my ideal body weight?** Gaining weight withouttrying is a sign of a poor diet. Following a healthy diet and getting regular exercise is the best way to lose weight and keep it off.

7. **Do I limit the amount of salt, sugar, alcohol and caffeine that I consume?**These are okay in moderation, but a lot of people use these in excessive amounts. These four elements can wreak havocon a healthy diet.

Variety – The Spice of Life

This saying is certainly true when it comes to eating a healthy diet. Many people get stuck in ruts where they eat too much of one type of food. This leaves their body with excessive nutrients in one area, and none in another. No one likes to eat the same thing everyday, but sometimes we do for the pure convenience of it.

There are a variety of foods that you can add to your diet to keep it from becoming stagnant and boring. There are hundreds of fruits and vegetables available at the average grocery store. There are also several other types of food that you can add to your diet including:

1. Fresh fruit
2. Vegetables
3. Meats
4. Whole grains

Variety is one of the things that nutritionists stress the most. They say that variety is important for both nutrition and psychological reasons. A varied diet is essential for a person to maintain good health and to maintain a good psychological well-being. Feeling deprived of your favorite foods can cause you to give up a healthy lifestyle. Variety allows you to incorporate your favorites with healthy foods and offers the chance for you to develop new favorites as well.

It is important that you continue to eat foods that you like, but in moderation. Instead of giving up bacon, have it as occasional treat. The same is true for desserts and sweets.

It is important that people eat from the five major food groups each day. TheUSDA identifies these food groups as:

1. Fresh fruit
2. Vegetables
3. Meats
4. Whole grains

By combining these food groups, you are ensuring that your body is receiving the necessary nutrients that these items contain. This helps to ensure properlevels of nutrition.

Simply eating from these groups is not enough. There are a variety of foods in these groups that would not necessarily be considered healthy such as ice cream or candied yams. The five food groups may be represented, but they don't do you much good if they are coated in sugar. Choosing the best foods from these groups is important as well.

Choosing healthy means that you want to look for foods that are not supped up with excess fat or sugar. It also means choosing meats from the lean section and removing the fat and skin from chicken. By doing this, you are eliminating unnecessary calories and excess fat.

When you choose breads and cereals, it is important not to choose those that are loaded with sugar or overly refined. Choose whole grains hat have not beenenhanced. Many of these whole grains are also fortified with additional vitamins and minerals. This insures that you are receiving these extra nutrients, but you should not rely on fortified foods alone. It is important that you get these nutrients in their natural form as well. Many foods are also supplemented with calcium and folic acid. These help to ensure that bones and teeth stay strong.

Folic acid is essential in preventing birth defects.

If you can substitute healthy foods for those that are less healthy, you will be on your way. For example, you can substitute skinless white meat chicken for darkmeat drumsticks. This is a good way to maximize nutrition without losing good food options.

Foods Working Together

It is important that you choose a combination of foods that provide you with optimum nutrition. This means combining foods such as meats, beans, dairy and vegetables and whole grains to form a well-rounded meal. All of these foods combined together will provide you with the different nutrients that your body needs.

Most foods are obviously healthy. However, it may be difficult to know whether some items are healthy or not. In this instance, you will want to look at the nutritional labels. Labels are required on all packaged foods and can be very helpful to those who are looking to eat a healthier diet. Not only do the labels tell you how many calories, fat grams and other nutritional information, but they also provide detailed information on the type of vitamins and minerals are in thefood as well.

When choosing healthy foods, small changes can make a big difference. Whenyou exchange fresh and low fat meals for high fat meals you will feel more energetic because you are not being "weighed down" by the high fat you were consuming in the past. You feel full without feeling bloated. You should also notice an increase in energy levels.

By replacing highly processed grains for nutritious whole grains you will find that you are consuming more nutrients. Many of your highly refined foods are stripped of the nutrients and they do you little good in terms of a healthy diet.

Cooking techniques are also important. It is imperative that you don't cook with high fat oil, but use a cooking spread instead. This ensures that you are not eating any unnecessary fats in the form of oil. If you cook vegetables too long, you may actually be cooking away significant amounts of nutrients. Take broccoli as an example. If you over boil it and then slather it in butter and cheese, you are cooking away nutrients and replacing them with fat. Boiling it too long can also cause them to lose nutrients. To prepare vegetables, you are often better off quickly steaming them in the microwave or over the stove. Cookthem in as little water as possible, but use enough to keep them from becoming scorched.

When you cook potatoes, it is a good idea to include the skin. The skin containsa lot of fiber, nutrients and minerals. You can also cook a baked potato in the microwave or grill to give it a better flavor. By using these methods, you will make the skin soft and minimize the need to load it with butter, sour cream, cheese, bacon, etc. In fact, healthier alternatives would include a little bit of nonfat cottage cheese or nonfat yogurt.

Chapter 2

Planning Healthy Meals

Planning healthy meals can be difficult, especially if you are cooking for a familywho is stuck in a rut of unhealthy meals. With some basic nutrition knowledge, however, you can have your family eating healthy without them really even realizing it.

The key to creating healthy meals is to plan. Plan your week's meals ahead of time and ensure you have all of the necessary ingredients. Don't put off preparing healthy meals because you don't have a tomato. Plan your meals out and go grocery shopping. While shopping it is important to get only the foods that are on your list and stay away from the cookie and ice cream aisles to limit temptation. This will also allow you to keep your food costs to a minimum because you are buying less expensive whole foods instead of processed foods.

Huge time savers such as slow cookers and microwaves are also helpful and everything that comes out of the microwave doesn't have to be unhealthy. A slow cooker will allow foods to cook all day while you are at work. When you get home, you have a delicious and healthy meal waiting for you.

On the weekends you can prepare meals ahead of time and put them in microwave safe dishes. When you have busy nights such as evenings that are full of sports games or practices with your children, all you have to do is pop their healthy meal into the microwave. There are several mircrowavable healthy meals that you can make at home and save for the rest of the week. These are also good if you are a single person living alone and have a hard time cooking for just one person. Divvy up the meals for the rest of the week.

When you are planning meals for the week, create a chart of each day's meals and your daily schedule. This will help you decide which days are best for certain meals. For example, maybe you have time to cook something extra special on Friday nights, but the rest of the week is so hectic you don't know if you are coming or going. You can place those special recipes you have been wanting to try on Friday and then come up with healthy alternatives for your busydays.

Getting the Family Involved

Eating healthy is a family affair. It is important to get your spouse and your kids involved. This allows you to ensure that each day someone has something that is his or her favorite being served. This may mean that Friday nights are special pizza nights, but the rest of the week is healthy. It is important to plan meals with everyone's input to ensure that everyone's tastes are involved. You also do not want anyone to feel as though they are being deprived of something they like.

It is an even better idea to get everyone involved in cooking. This allows the children to learn their way around the kitchen and what foods are healthy for them to eat.

Get Prepared

Cooking in large quantities is an excellent way for you to have healthy foods at your fingertips. Cooking large amounts of soups, casseroles, chilies and pasta will save you a lot of time during the week. You can even make double or triplebatches of certain staples in your diet. This will allow you to freeze them and use them later. This saves you both time and money.

When you freeze your leftovers, be sure that you label your containers with freezer tape and permanent marker. This will allow you to rotate items wisely and keep the older foods near the top. This also allows you to avoid waste by not having to throw out foods that have expired.

Stock up on meats when they are on sale and then divide them up into individual serving portions for your family. For example, if you buy 5 pounds of ground beef, separate it out into 5 one-pound servings for your ground beef recipes.

You can also divide up your chicken breasts, turkey, steaks, roasts and pork chops. If you are going to have pork chops one night, all you have to do is pull them out of the freezer and allow them to thaw while you are at work. When you get home you can cook them up on the grill and sauté up some fresh veggies.

A well-stocked pantry is also important. Keep a good supply of the staples such as canned veggies, fruits, soup stocks, etc. These will help you prepare your meals much more quickly, especially when combined with your stocked freezer. This also allows you to save time and money.

Other items that you can stock up on include:

1. Whole grain cereals
2. Pastas
3. Tomato sauce
4. Baked beans
5. Canned salmon
6. Tuna

7. Whole grain breads

Eating for Maximum Nutrition

In the past several years there have been a lot of fad diets hit the market. This is mainly because people are recognizing that it is time to start eating better and living a more healthy lifestyle. We all know that you need to eat fruits and vegetables, but we are far too often choosing the wrong items. For example, avocados may look like a healthy food, but they are actually full of fat and calories. Bananas may seem healthy, but they have a lot of sugar. It is the healthy balance of these items that we are looking for.

The key to changing your diet is to recognize the areas that you need to changeand then work on those areas. For instance, some people simply need to add veggies to their diet and cut back on meats. Others need to cut back on sweets and add fruits and vegetables. Some people could do themselves a lot of good by eating a breakfast so that they do not overeat later in the day. These are littlechanges that can be made if you get motivated to do it. The key is to make small changes so that they are seamlessly incorporated into your life.

Eating healthy also means different things to different people. A healthy runner who runs a 5K every other weekend doesn't have the same nutritional requirements as an office worker who sits at a desk all day and needs to lose 20pounds.

A good place to start is to begin by changing your diet up by adding variety. Make smarter choices when shopping and try to avoid the sugary temptations that lurk in the grocery store. If you eat out a lot, you can still make better choices. Limit your salad dressing and eat more veggies and skinless chicken. It is also a good idea not to eat your whole plate but to take a portion of it homewith you for later.

Eat more highly nutritious foods rather than high calorie foods. You will be amazed at the difference this can make at your first sitting. Most fatty foods are full of empty calories. This means you are eating foods that have a lot of calories but they don't fill you up. By eating foods that have calories you use, you are feeding yourself useful energy without overeating on unhealthy foods. The produce section of the grocery store contains a lot of healthy and filling foods that are not full of empty calories.

Don't be afraid to try new things. Your tastes change as you grow older. You actually begin to like foods that you despised as a child. Some people think that they don't like foods, but they have never eaten many of what they say they don't like. Produce is relatively cheap. So you are not losing too much money if you by some fresh spinach for a salad and find out you still don't like it. If you do likeit, then you found something healthy that you don't mind eating and it's relatively inexpensive. Talk about a win-win situation!

You don't have to give up your Saturday night steak. Just work on it a bit to make it healthier. Cut off the excess fat that you don't need and don't slatheryour potato in all the "fixins." Try a little bit of butter or even a little cottage cheese.

Healthy Snacks

It never fails, there's a pang that hits our stomach around 2:30 or 3:00 in theafternoon. This little bit of hunger is easily overcome by a healthy snack.

Instead of reaching for those chocolate chip cookies, why not some apple wedges with a little peanut butter on them? Or, how about a glass of milk or cupof cottage cheese? You could even grab a handful of nuts. Whole grain products make good snacks as well. Wheat bread or bagels can make you a nice little snack to hold you over until dinner.

For the kids, consider having some carrot sticks already peeled and sliced for them when they come home from school. You could even have a little bowl of broccoli florets, green peppers and carrots in a bowl with a little side of low fatsalad dressing for dipping. These are much better snacks than Jell-O, Fruit Roll-Ups, Pop Tarts or candy bars.

Here is a little quick recipe that you can whip up in no time:

1. Can of mandarin oranges
2. Cut up banana
3. Apple
4. Nectarine
5. Strawberries
6. Blueberries
7. Raisins

Mix in the juices from the orange and serve. This is a delicious little fresh fruit salad that you can use as a snack or even a healthy dessert.

Keeping a bowl of fresh fruit around on the table also encourages you to grab an apple or orange instead of a handful of M&Ms.

Milk and dairy products are also important. You don't have to buy the fattiest of these items either. If you are a whole milk drinker, consider dropping down to 2%. You will be amazed that the taste is very similar to whole milk, but with less fat. It is also not as watery as skim milk. You can also have some low-fat or nonfat yogurt, puddings, cheeses and cottage cheese around.

Lunchmeats can also make a great snack. Get some healthy turkey, chicken orham. Pregnant women should be sure to warm these up to kill off any bacteria before eating them, just to be on the safe side. Sandwiches that are made on whole grain bread with low calorie mustard can be a good snack to hold you over.

Tuna that is packed in water is the best and very easy to whip up. Peanutbutter, eggs, poultry, nuts and beans make good snacks as well.

You can also pair your fresh fruit with nonfat plain or vanilla yogurt. Add fruit tocereal or use fresh fruit and juices to make smoothies as a quick snack or breakfast.

For bagels that are getting a little stale, toast them and spread a little bit of peanut butter on them. You could also use a low fat cream cheese. Or, slice them into little thin slices and brush with a little butter. Sprinkle with a little garlicand bake for 10-12 minutes at 350 degrees. Now you have healthy bagel chips and you didn't waste any food.

Taking Your Lunch With You

When you are a career person, it can be difficult not to eat out everyday for lunch. It is possible to take your healthy lifestyle on the go. You also neverknow what they are serving in school cafeterias these days, especially when it comes to older kids in middle school or high school. If you all brown bag it, then you can still create healthy lunches for your whole family.

The most important decision to make is what you are putting in those lunchboxes. It is very important that you choose foods that are easy, yet quick. If you are able to include a favorite food in each lunch, then there isless of a chance of your child hitting a vending machine to get a candy bar.

When you are packing lunches, be sure to choose at least three of the following:

1. 1 fruit or vegetable (fresh, canned or frozen)
2. Whole grain product
3. Milk or dairy production
4. Meat, fish, poultry, eggs, peanut butter, legumes or hummus

It is also a good idea to get the family involved in fixing their lunches. Have a little session each night where everyone gets to choose some of these healthy items to put in their lunches. Lie out all of the healthy food options and let everyone decide what they want to take with them the next day. If they want milkto drink, it is a good idea to give them milk money, as it is difficult to keep milk cold at school.

Kids will love to fix their own lunches. You might even have a special shelf in the refrigerator just for those foods. It is also a good idea to have plastic bags, napkins, plastic silverware and straws for the kids to pack in their lunches aswell.

Healthy Lunch Tips

1. Incorporate different breads in sandwiches.
    - Rye
    - Pumpernickel
    - Whole Wheat
    - Tortilla wraps
    - Pitas
    - Bread sticks
    - Crackers
2. Bite sized veggies are best
    - Baby carrots
    - Broccoli florets
    - Pepper slices
3. Bite sized fruit are good too
    - Grapes
    - Blueberries
    - Orange wedges
    - Strawberries
4. 100% fruit juice or milk money
5. Single serving cereals (Good for breakfast too)
6. Selection of various nonfat yogurts.

Chapter 3

Understanding Nutrition

There are numerous nutrients that make up our diet. Each nutrient plays an important role in our diet and our diet is not well rounded without all of them. The basic building blocks to a healthy diet include:

1. Carbohydrates
2. Protein
3. Fats
4. Vitamins
5. Minerals

Fats

Fats and carbohydrates make up a healthy diet. The key is to not to overeat either one of these to the point that they are not healthy for you. Many peopledo not understand the role that fats and carbs play in our diet. While these should be limited, they are still important for a healthy lifestyle. The key is to make smart decisions when it comes to choosing which fats and oils you are going to eat. This means that you will want to substitute saturated fats with unsaturated fats. You want to cook with lighter oils when cooking.

Fats are essential for supplying the body with energy. Fats are essential so that fatty acids and aid in the transportation of fat-soluble vitamins around the body. These fat-soluble vitamins include:

1. Vitamin A
2. Vitamin D
3. Vitamin E
4. Vitamin K
5. Carotenoids

Fats are also the building blocks for many tissues and membranes. They play many roles in regulating the various bodily functions.

Dietary fat is available in both plant and animal sources of food. Many nutrition experts recommend that the intake of fat should be kept to less than 20% of calories. Extreme low fat diets, however, are not safe and cause damage to thebody.

The type of fat that you take in also makes a huge difference. A diet that is high in saturated fats, cholesterol and trans fats have been associated with numerous conditions including:

1. Heart disease
2. Heart attacks
3. Stroke
4. Chronic health problems
5. Diabetes
6. Obesity

Excessive fat intake of saturated fats and trans fats are associated with the greatest complications. Trans fats are those fats that are solid at room temperature. One of the best ways to limit the intake of saturated fat is to limitthe intake of animal fat in the diet. Animal fats include meats such as:

1. Bacon
2. Sausage
3. Butter
4. Ice cream

Cholesterol can be regulated by watching the intake of eggs and organ meats, as well as other foods that are known to be high in cholesterol.

Food labels can make it difficult to determine which fats are good fats. forexample, trans fats are listed on the ingredient lists and not in the chart of dietary information. Processed foods contain more trans fats.

Polyunsaturated and monounsaturated fats are better choices. These can be found in canola and olive oil. These are lighter oils and it is a big step towards healthier eating if you incorporate these into your diet instead of using fats such as lard to cook with. These fats are liquid at room temperature. They also haveheart-protecting qualities, unlike trans fats.

Fish also contain good fats. They are a source of omega-3 fatty acids. Thesehave been found to help lower cholesterol and to promote good health. They

Carbohydrates

These are important of a healthy diet, although the marketing of some diets mayhave you think otherwise. They are necessary for providing your with energy as well as essential nutrients. Carbohydrates are found in a variety of foods including fruits, vegetables, grains and dairy products. They are not all equally healthy, so it is important that you choose wisely.

When you are choosing your breads and cereals, look to have them made with whole grains. While avoiding the more highly refined varieties. It is also important to limit the intake of sugars, such as baked goods and candy.

Consuming large amounts of these low nutrient and high calorie foods can makeit difficult to stay healthy without gaining weight.

Many people consume way too much sugar and salt. Salt is important in nutrition, but many people consume too much of it. Excess salt causes water retention, high blood pressure and other conditions. Choose low sodium foodsand limit the use of the saltshaker. By implementing these two strategies, you will be able to go a long way.

Carbohydrates are found in a lot of foods. For instance, cookies and whole wheat bread are both sources of carbohydrates. Whole wheat bread is much more healthy than cookies. This is where the importance of good decisions comes into play.

In addition to cereals and breads, carbohydrates are also present in fruits and vegetables. They are also available in dairy products. Carbohydrates and fatsalso help to provide variety in the diet.

When it comes to choosing carbohydrates it is best to choose those that are not refined. When carbs enter the small intestine they are broken down into sugars.Those carbs that are from refined products are broken down into sugar much more quickly.

Antioxidants

There has been a lot of talk lately about how antioxidants are important in the diet. They have a possible role in fighting a variety of illnesses and this includessome types of cancer. They are also supposed to aid in age related degeneration and heart disease.

Many companies are marketing various pills, powders and capsules. The marketing of these supplements stresses that you need you supplement yourdiet in this pill form, however it is best to receive these nutrients through everyday foods and not from supplements.

It is important to understand how antioxidants work to protect the body. Antioxidants work to neutralize harmful elements that are known as free radicals.These are produced in the body naturally and as a consequence of natural bodily processes. Most of the time the body will be able to neutralize and eliminate free radicals on its own.

Stresses such as environmental pollution, a weak immune system, UV radiation and alcohol cause the body to not be able to effectively fight these free radicals.Excessive free radicals in the human body can cause damage to the structure and function of the various organs and other systems in the body. Recent studies have also shown free radicals cause a number of diseases. They may also play a role in aging.

It is estimated that foods have about 4,000 different compounds that have antioxidant qualities. Since only a small number of these compounds have beenidentified it is difficult to see why adding a supplement would help achieve a healthy diet. You are better off eating a variety of foods and receiving antioxidants the natural way.

There are many sources of antioxidant vitamins including:

Vitamin C: This is probably the most studied of all the antioxidant vitamins. It isalso known as ascorbic acid. Vitamin C is believed to be the body's first line of defense against infection and disease. Vitamin C is water-soluble and must be consumed daily. It is available in:

1. Grapefruit
2. Green peppers
3. Broccoli
4. Leafy greens
5. Strawberries
6. Cabbage
7. Potatoes

Vitamin E: This is a fat-soluble vitamin that is stored in the liver and other tissues. It has been studied for its effect on aging and healing sunburns. It is important that your diet contains adequate amounts of vitamin E. Vitamin E canbe found in:

1. Whole wheat germ
2. Nuts
3. Seeds
4. Whole grains
5. Vegetable oil
6. Fish liver oil
7. Leafy greens

Beta-carotene: This is the nutrient that causes flamingos to be pink, as the receive it from the shrimp that they eat. There are over 600 carotenoids that have been discovered so far. The role of beta-carotene in nature is to protect the skins of fruits that are dark green, yellow and orange. Beta-carotene can be found in:

1. Carrots
2. Squash
3. Sweet potatoes
4. Broccoli
5. Tomatoes
6. Collard greens
7. Kale
8. Cantaloupe
9. Peaches10 Apricots

Selenium: This is one of the most important minerals in a healthy diet. It hasproperties that prevent cell damage, which is seen as an important part of preventing cancer. It is important to get selenium naturally from your diet, as supplements can be toxic. It is easily found in foods such as:

1. Fish
2. Shellfish
3. Red meat
4. Whole grains

5. Poultry
6. Eggs
7. Garlic
8. Vegetables that have been grown in selenium rich soils

Choosing Low Fat and High Fiber Foods

Raising the level of dietary fiber is important. At the same time it is important to lower the amount of fat in your diet. Adding dietary fiber to your diet is one of the most effective changes that you can make. However, many people consume way too much fat without enough fiber.

A good place to start is by knowing which foods you eat are high in fiber or which foods that are high in fiber that you could eat. Eating a diet that is rich in fiber will lower fat and other negative diet elements.

When you are boosting the amount of fiber in your diet you also want to do so ata gradual rate. Abrupt changes in fiber can cause abdominal pain, cramps, bloating and gas.

There are several high fiber foods including:

1. Dried peas & beans
2. Dried fruits
3. Nuts

4. Sesame seeds
5. Sunflower seeds
6. Berries

All of these foods have more than 6 grams of fiber per serving.

Foods which contain 4 to 6 grams of fiber per serving include:

1. Baked potatoes with skin
2. Apples
3. Pears
4. Barley
5. Brown rice
6. Bran muffins
7. Lima beans
8. Snow peas
9. Green peas
10. Sweet potatoes

Foods that contain 2 to 4 grams per serving include:

1. Vegetables
2. Citrus fruits
3. Whole wheat bread

4. Rye bread
5. Melons

You will need to eat more of these foods to get the full effect, but that is okaybecause they are nutritious foods.

In order to have healthier eating habits for life, it is important to change the way you shop, cook and eat. A diet change should be something that you intend to continue with through life, so it is important that you develop good habits now that will allow you to do so.

When you go grocery shopping, get into the habit of hitting the produce sectionfirst. This is generally easy because most grocery stores have it conveniently located near the front door. You will want to purchase fresh fruits and vegetables that are in season. These foods contain rich sources of vitamins and minerals. They also have a lot of fiber. Canned fruits and vegetables are okay if they are not in season.

When you are looking at baked goods, try to find those that are made with:

1. Whole wheat flour
2. Wheat bran
3. Oat bran
4. Poppy seeds

5. Sesame seeds
6. Oatmeal
7. Raisins

It is also important that you learn to read labels. There are federally mandated labels on all foods that are sold. These labels are also standardized and contain certain information. Look at:

1. Calorie content
2. Fiber content
3. Vitamin content

You can also find this information on meats, seafood and poultry as well.

Fiber Myths

There are several myths about fiber. The first is that the crispness of a food is related to fiber. The truth is that there is no relation here. The amount of crispness of a food product does not indicate the amount of fiber that the product contains. The crunch of lettuce, for example, is from the amount of water that it contains.

Secondly, many people think that cooking breaks down fiber. This is not true either. Cooking has no effect on the amount of fiber that the food contains.

Peeling vegetables and fruits, however, will remove some fiber since the skins contain fiber. Edible skins, such as apple peel, are a good source of fiber.

No matter why you need to increase your fiber intake, you will find that it is a positive change to make in your diet. Increasing the amount of fiber you receive can have a large impact on your health.

Understanding Portion Sizes

We have all heard the USDA report that we need to eat 5 to 10 servings of fruit and vegetables each day. This is really confusing because that sounds like a whole lot of food. Exactly what is a serving?

A serving a fruit or vegetable may be:

1. A medium sized piece of fruit
2. One large slice of fruit
3. Two pieces of small fruit
4. 1 cup strawberries, raspberries or grapes
5. ½ cup of fresh fruit salad

6. ½ cup of stewed or canned fruit
7. ¼ cup of dried fruit
8. ½ cup of 100% pure fruit juice
9. ½ cup of cooked, canned or frozen vegetables10 1 side salad

Unlike other foods, the more the better when it comes to eating fruits and vegetables. Be sure to include as many servings of fruits and vegetables as youcan when planning your meals.

Tips for Healthier Living

1. Stock your fridge with celery or carrots
2. Keep a bowl of fruits ready to be eaten out on the table or kitchencounter
3. Eat warm vegetable soup on a cold day
4. Eat at least one salad per day
5. Snack on apples and oranges or dried fruits
6. Add sprouts, cucumbers, lettuce and tomatoes to sandwiches forvariety.
7. Garnish meals with grated or chopped carrots
8. Eat two servings of veggies with each dinner
9. Try vegetable stir fry

10. Make vegetable kabobs on the grill

11. Use baked apples or pears for dessert

12. Add veggies such as carrots, cabbage, onions, lentils and peas tosoups, stews and casseroles.

Tips for Choosing Fruits and Vegetables

1. When possible, choose fresh fruits. Fresh fruits and vegetablescontain more nutrients than frozen or dried varieties.

2. Frozen and canned vegetables are good for those fruits andvegetables that are out of season.

3. Choose fruits and vegetables from a variety of different colors.

4. Be careful when cooking vegetables.

5. Keep your vegetables healthy by adding minimal butter, margarineand oil.

6. Be careful when cooking vegetables. It is best to quick steam in themicrowave with minimal water.

Get Fishy in Your Diet

Fish allows you to maximize protein while keeping the fat and calories low. Thisis why fish is great for those people who are trying to lose weight and enjoy a healthier diet. There are very few foods that are capable of combing low fat and low calories, and then have high protein. High protein usually comes with high fat and high calories.

Many people are leery of fish because they have had fish that is not very fresh. Other people are leery because they don't know how to cook it. Fish dishes canseem challenging but they are actually quite easy. The amount of protein in fresh and frozen fish and seafood is very high. It is much higher than sources such as beef, pork and lamb.

CPSIA information can be obtained
at www.ICGtesting.com
Printed in the USA
LVHW081926271122
734044LV00013BA/581